The Gift

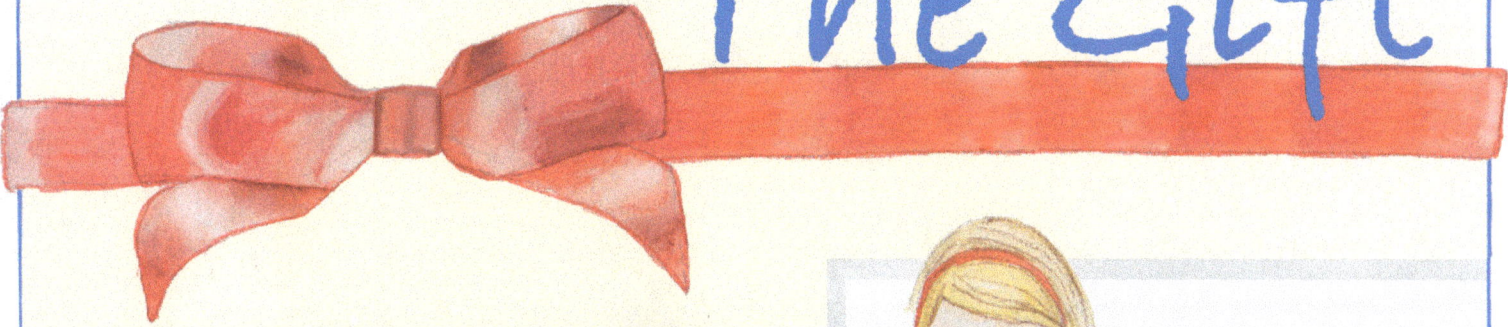

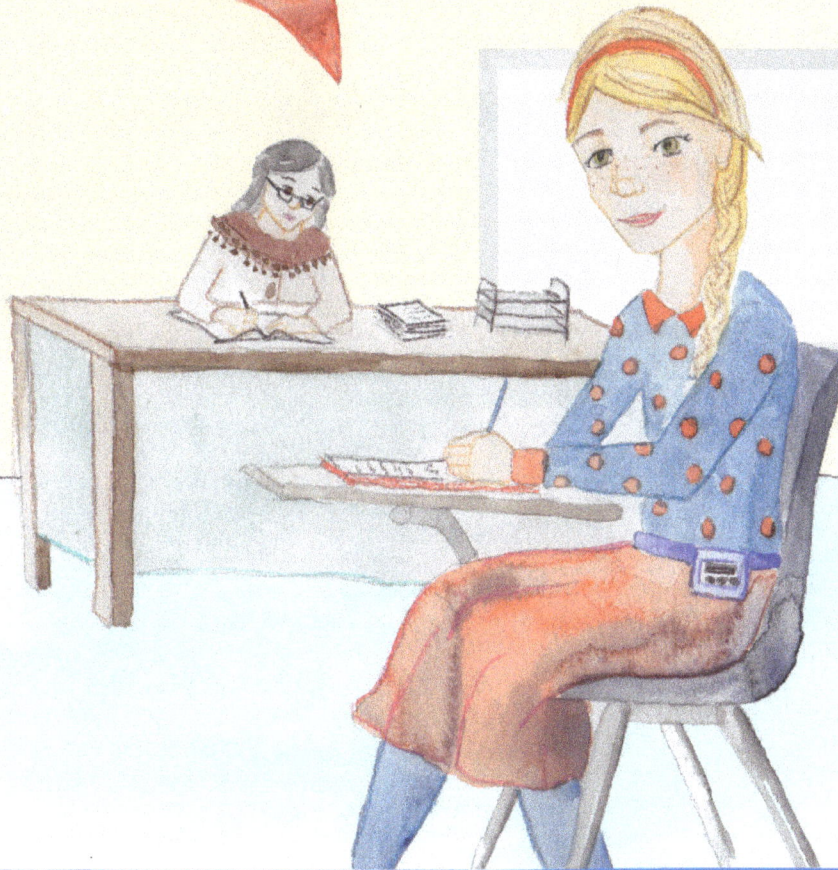

written by
Joseph J Swope

illustrations by
Chandra Swope

ISBN: 978-1-61296-586-4

PUBLISHED BY BLACK ROSE WRITING

www.blackrosewriting.com

Suggested Retail Price $12.95

The Gift is printed in Neutra Text Expert

Dedicated to my wife, Selena, who has bravely battled diabetes for many years. Her real life incident while attending nursing school served as the inspiration for this story.

A portion of the proceeds from this book will be donated to the JDRF.

Nearly two million people are diagnosed with diabetes each year in the United States. One person is identified with a new case of diabetes every 30 seconds.

Samantha – or Sam for short – was in many ways a typical eight-year-old girl. She collected dolls, played on the school soccer team, and liked to dabble with makeup.

But Sam was different from most girls her age in one important way. She had Type 1 diabetes.

Diabetes is a disease that doesn't allow people to control the amount of sugar in their blood. Samantha had diabetes since she was very young. If she didn't care for her diabetes, the disease could cause many serious health problems.

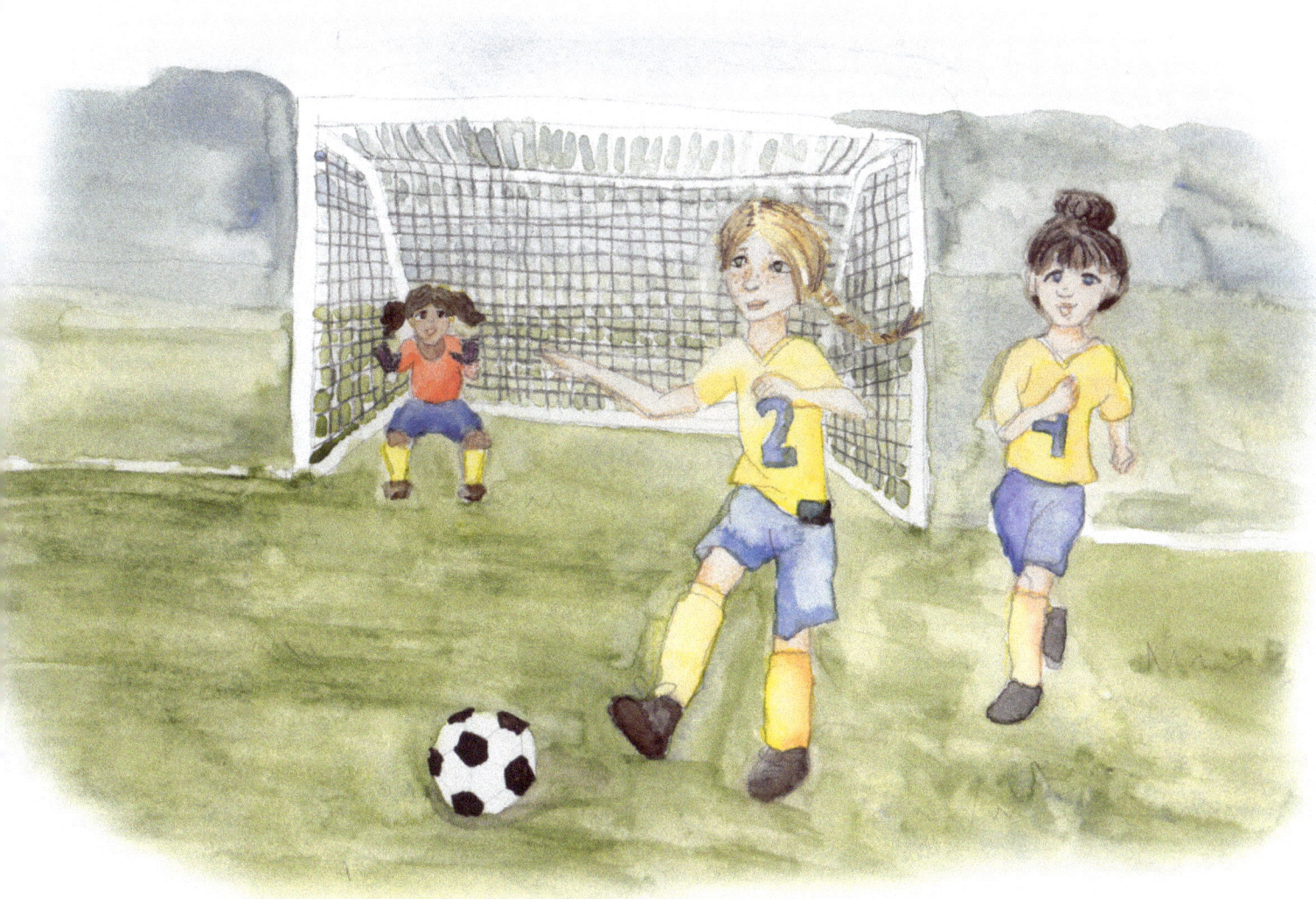

So every morning, when Samantha got dressed for school, she remembered to clip her insulin pump to her clothes. Insulin is a drug that helps diabetics control their blood sugar. Many children and adults wear pumps that deliver insulin automatically throughout the day.

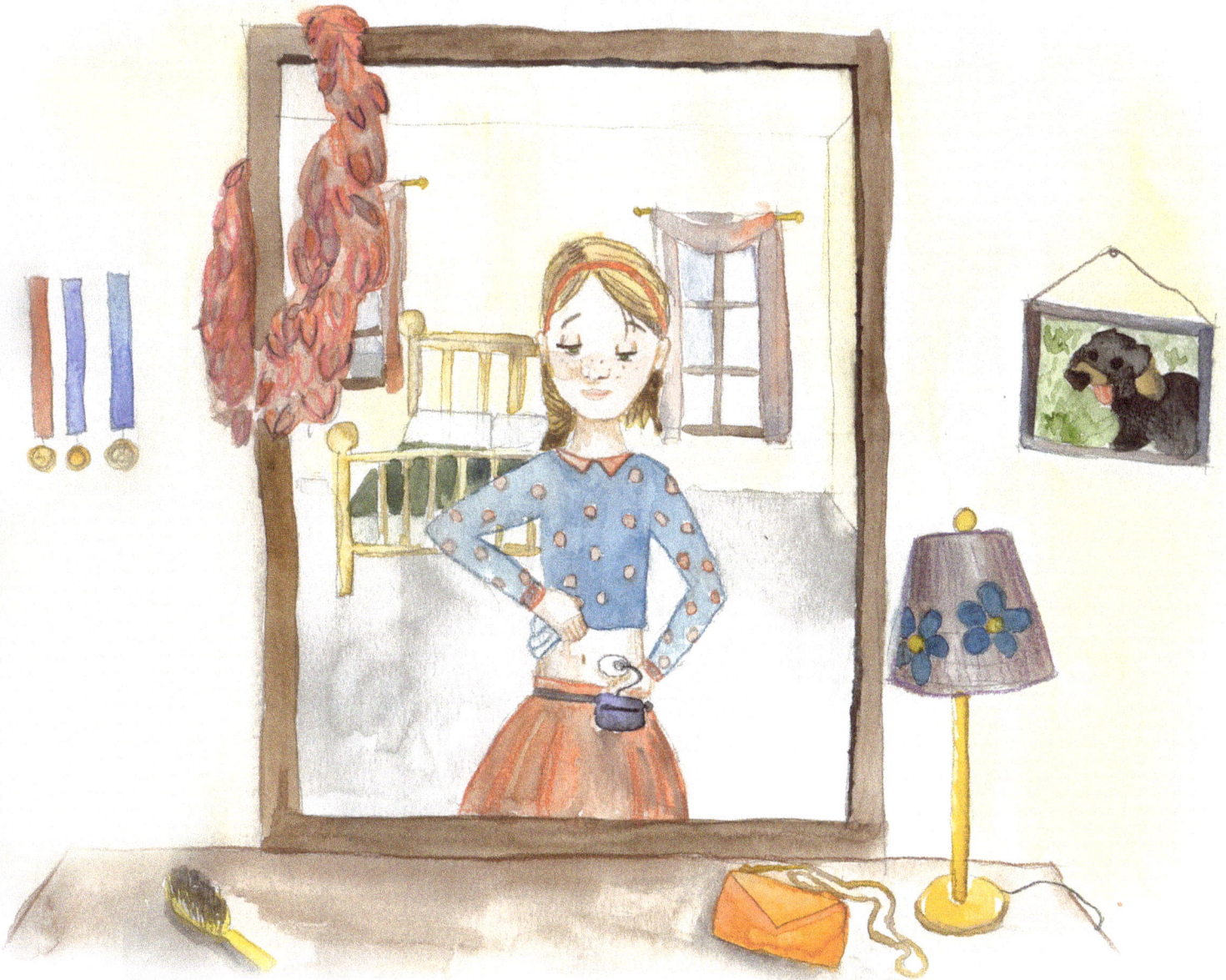

After she finished getting dressed, Sam ran downstairs and ate a healthy breakfast. Then her parents made sure she had her book bag all packed before she left for school.

"I love you, Mommy and Daddy," she said to her parents, giving each a quick kiss.

"We love you too," her mother said. "Have a good day in school."

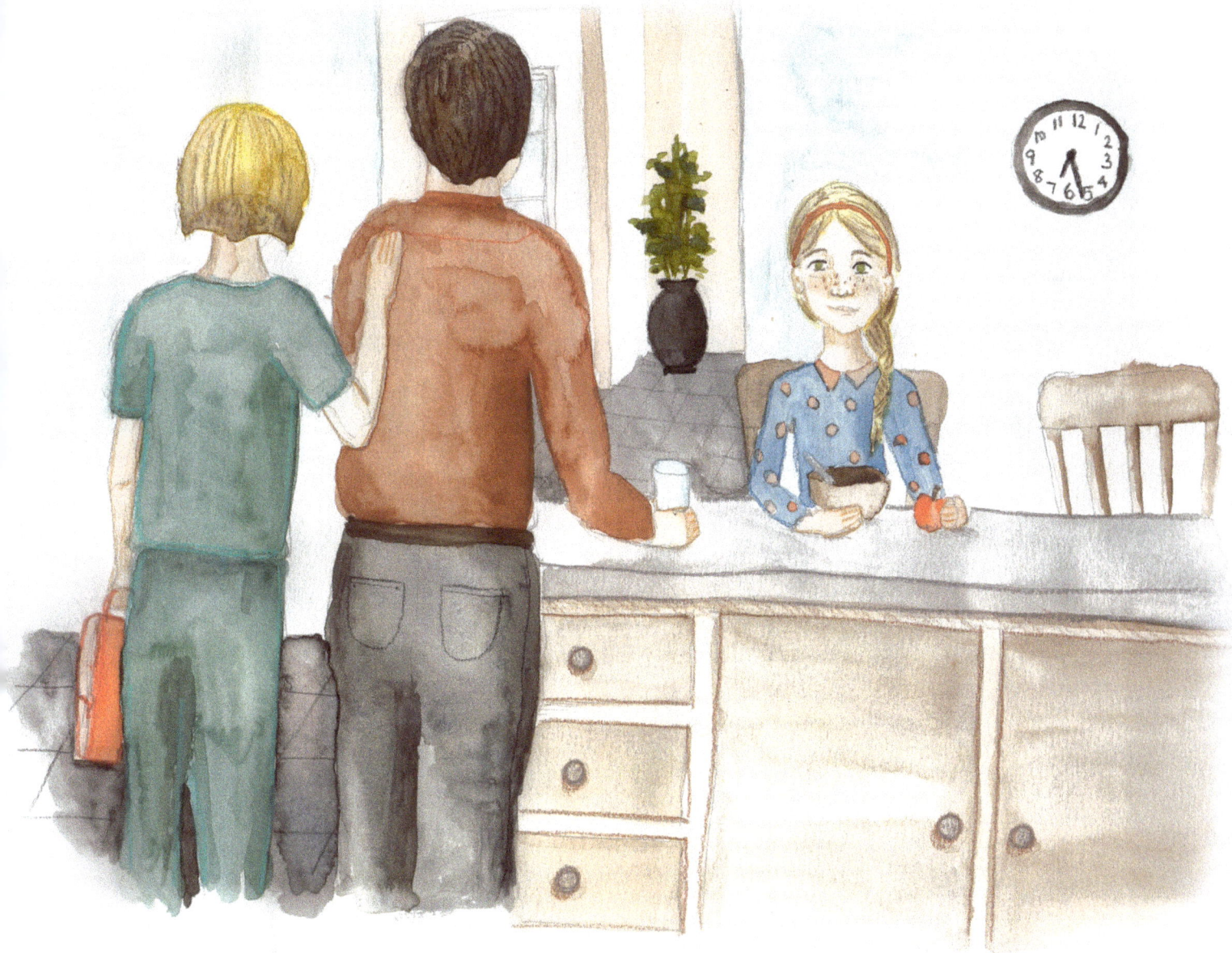

Samantha met several of her friends and together, the girls walked to school. In a few minutes, the third-graders reached room 217 and greeted their teacher, Mrs. Hunter.

"Good morning, Sam," Mrs. Hunter said. "Don't you look all dressed up today?"

Samantha looked down at the colorful dress and leggings she wore that day. "It's my favorite outfit," she said.

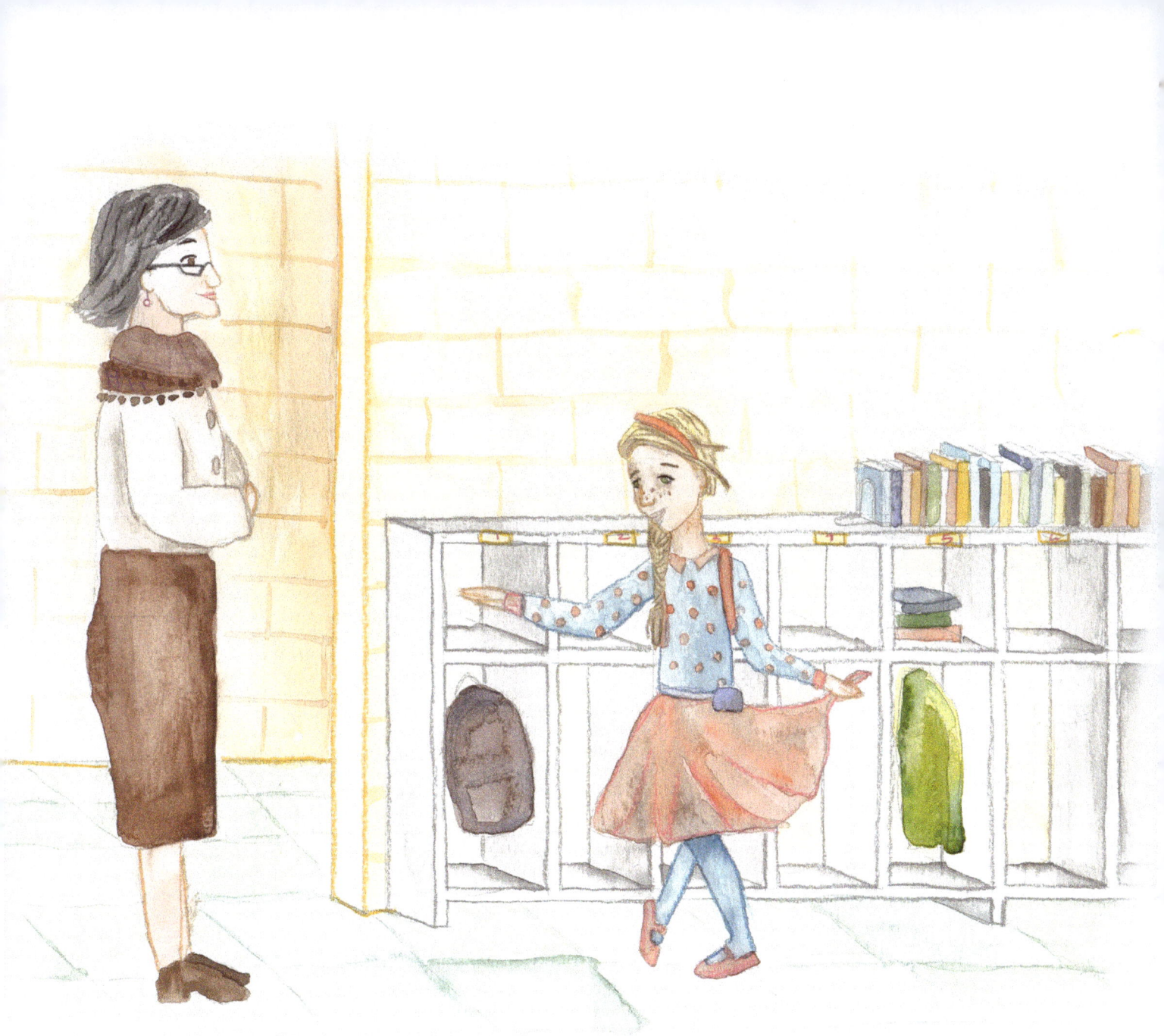

Samantha and her classmates had a busy day at school, studying mathematics, reading and science. Sam's favorite topic was reading, and she enjoyed turning verbs into past tense during class.

Sam noticed that Mrs. Hunter looked tired and not herself, but her teacher never complained.

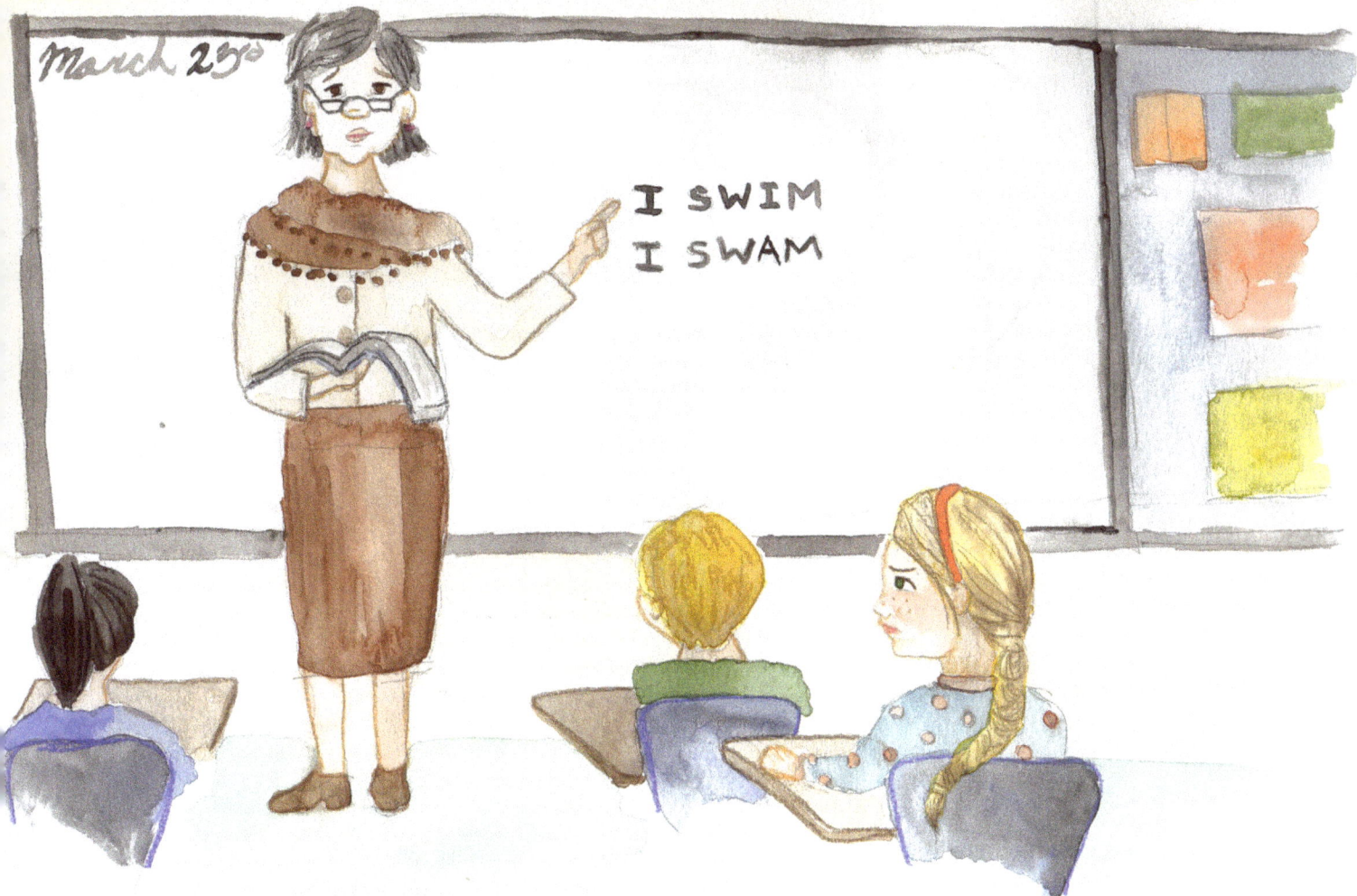

March 23rd

Aa Bb Cc Dd Ee Ff Gg Hh Ii Jj Kk Ll Mm Nn Oo Pp Qq Rr Ss Tt Uu

I SWIM
I SWAM

At lunch, Sam ordered a toasted cheese sandwich, tomato soup and an apple, along with milk to drink. Sam and her friends were talking about their upcoming soccer game on Saturday when Mrs. Hunter came to their table and sat down to chat with them.

Sam's teacher looked flush and she carried a large container of iced tea with her. As soon as she sat down, Mrs. Hunter drank the entire carton in two large gulps.

"I don't know what is the matter with me lately," Mrs. Hunter said to her students. "I've been so thirsty."

Sam looked at her teacher with concern.

"How long have you felt like this?" the eight-year-old asked.

"It's been a couple of weeks," Mrs. Hunter admitted. "I'm always tired and I'm drinking all the time."

11

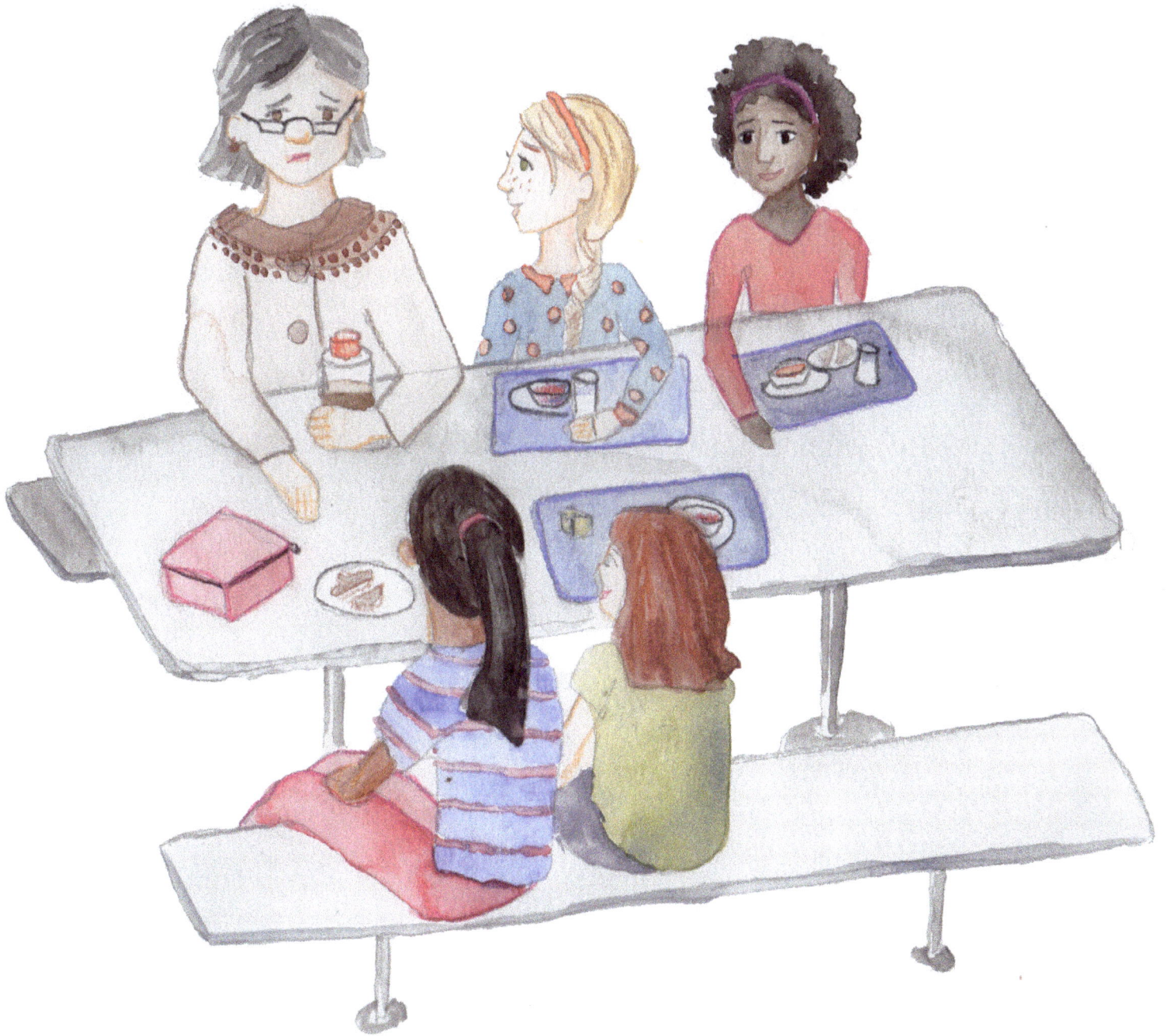

Sam opened up the small purse she always carried with her.

"Do you mind if I test your blood sugar?" she asked.

Mrs. Hunter looked at her student quizzically. "Why would you want to do that?"

"How you're feeling is a lot like I feel when my sugar is high," Sam explained. "It doesn't hurt to test it and make sure everything is OK."

Mrs. Hunter hesitated for a moment, but could see how concerned her student appeared. "Sure," the teacher finally concluded. "I've never had my blood sugar tested."

"I'll be gentle," Sam assured her.

Sam walked over to the first aid station and picked out a pair of latex gloves, just as she was taught to do in class. She carefully slipped the gloves over both hands. "They're a little big," she said. "But I can work with them."

Sam pulled out her diabetic equipment from her purse. She carefully took out a new lancet and inserted it into her lancing device. Then, she pulled out a test strip and prepared her glucometer to check the level of Mrs. Hunter's sugar in her blood. Sam knew a normal reading would be between 80 and 100.

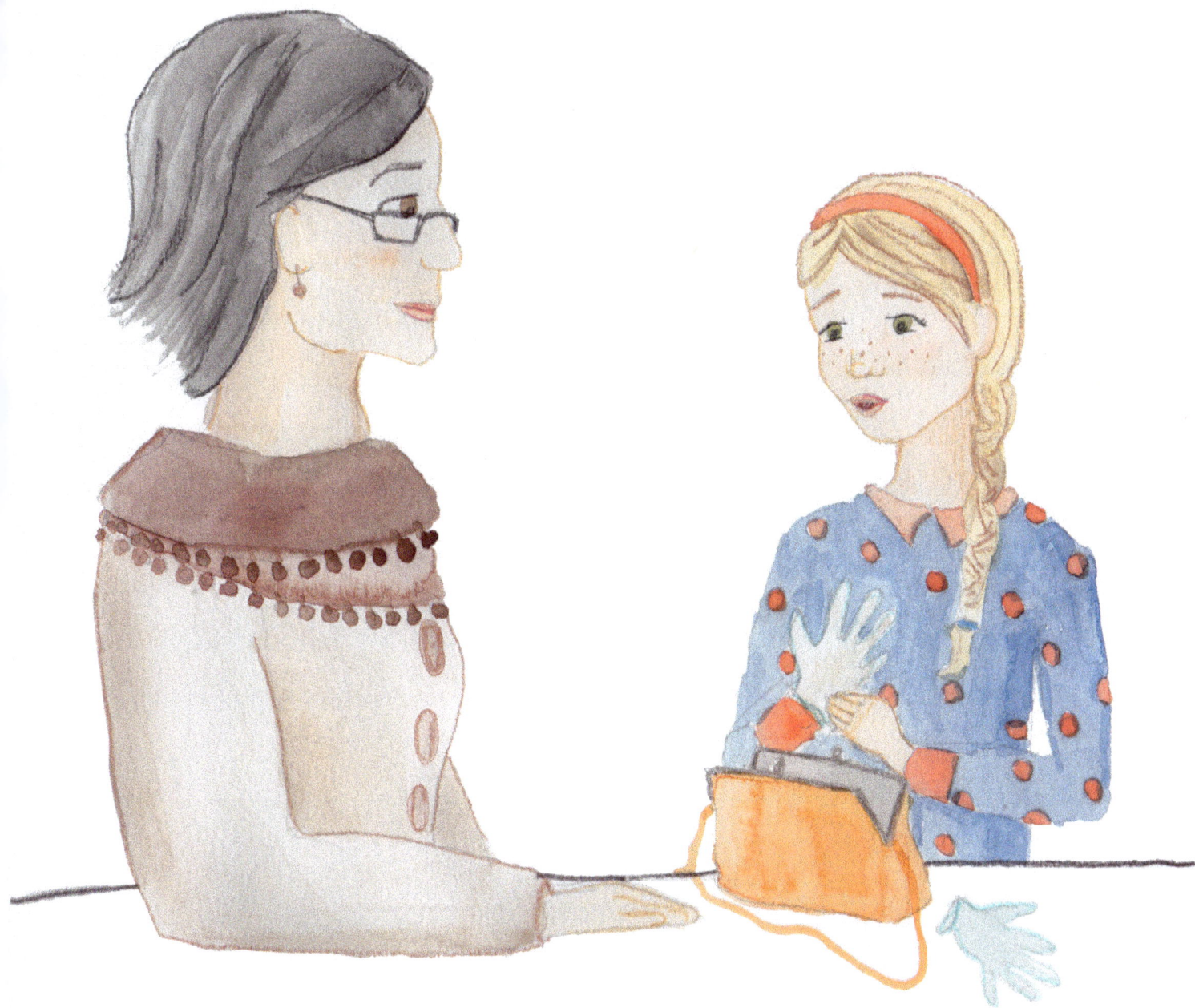

As gently as she could, Sam pricked Mrs. Hunter's finger with the lancet and drew a small drop of blood. Sam carefully lifted the blood onto the test strip and inserted it into the glucometer.

The glucometer counted down as it analyzed the blood. 5. . .4. . .3. . .2. . .1. . .

It read "438."

"That can't be right," Sam said. "Did you have sugar on your finger from anything you ate?"

"I don't know," Mrs. Hunter admitted. "Let me wash my hands and we'll try again."

After Mrs. Hunter washed her hands thoroughly, Sam went through the same careful steps and tested a finger on her teacher's other hand. Mrs. Hunter's blood sugar again read over 400.

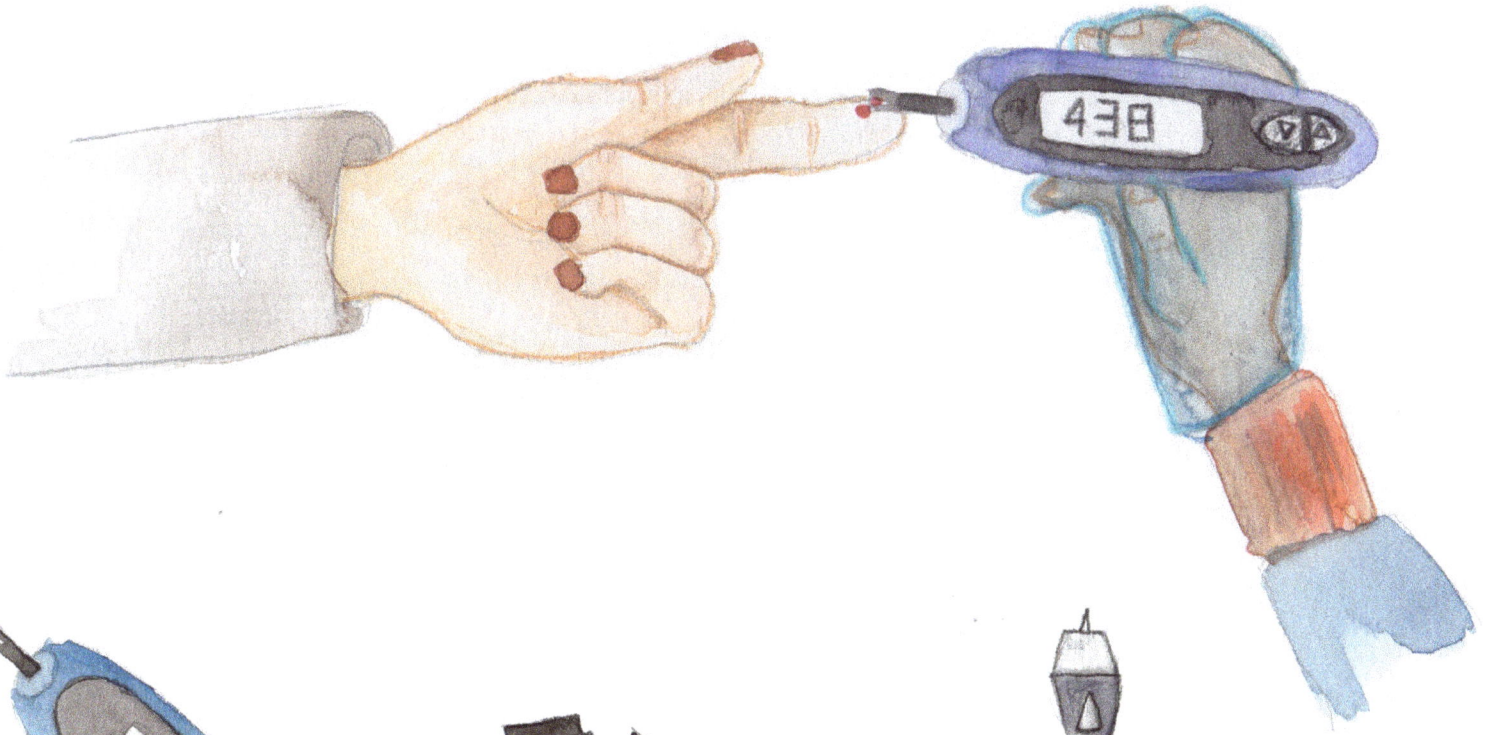

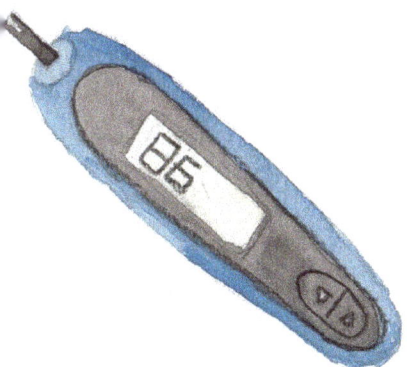

GLUCOMETER

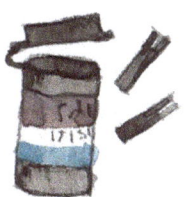

TEST STRIPS

LANCET

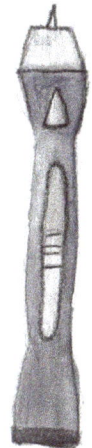

LANCET PEN

"I think you might want to see the nurse," Sam said to her teacher.

"I think you're right," Mrs. Hunter agreed.

Sam's teacher was admitted into the hospital later that day and stayed several days as doctors and nurses worked to bring her blood sugar under control.

Mrs. Hunter was diagnosed with Type 2 diabetes, a form of the disease that typically affects adults. She spent many hours learning about the medications needed to control her blood sugar, proper diet and warning signs that her blood sugar may be high or low.

When Mrs. Hunter returned to school the next week, she pulled Sam aside.

"Thank you, Sam," the teacher said. "You gave me a wonderful gift. You saved my life."

Sam smiled. "Diabetes is a terrible disease," she told her teacher. "You can never get away from it. But maybe that's why I have it - to help someone who didn't realize they needed it."

17

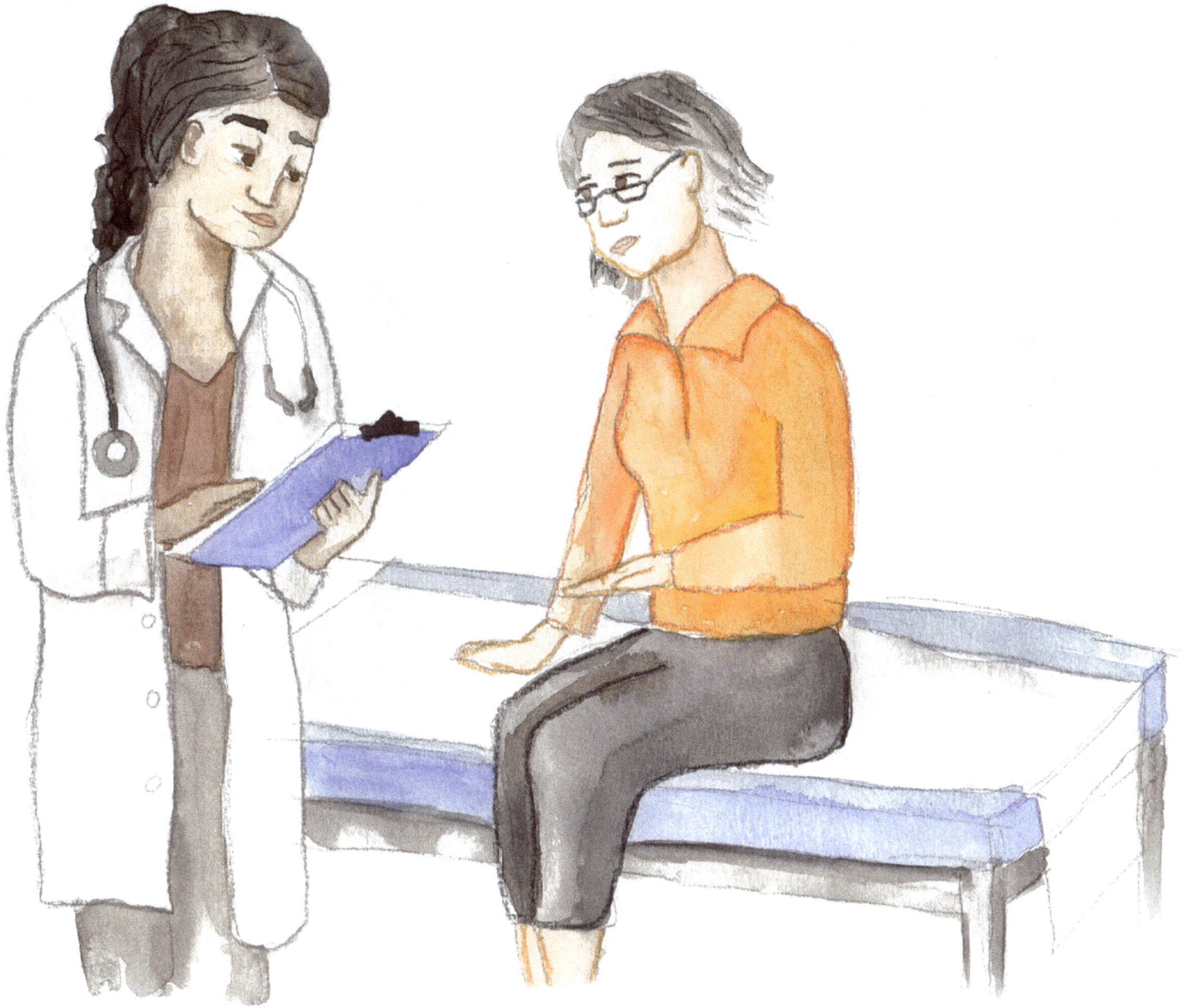

Mrs. Hunter smiled. "Maybe so," she agreed. "You're awfully wise for an eight-year-old."

"Maybe one day I'll become a doctor who helps lots of people with diabetes," Samantha said. "Maybe I'll even find a cure."

"You would be a very good doctor," Mrs. Hunter said. "If you do become a doctor, I hope you do find a cure! That would be wonderful!"

Together, the teacher and her student returned to their classroom.

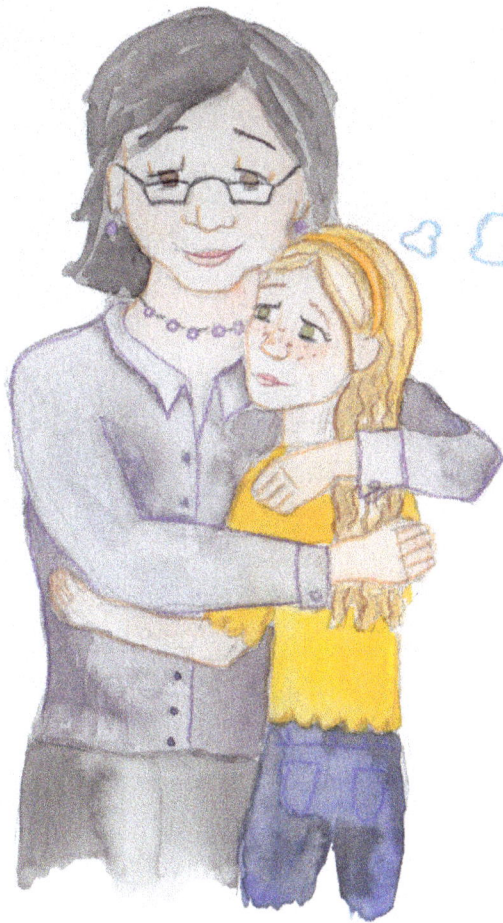
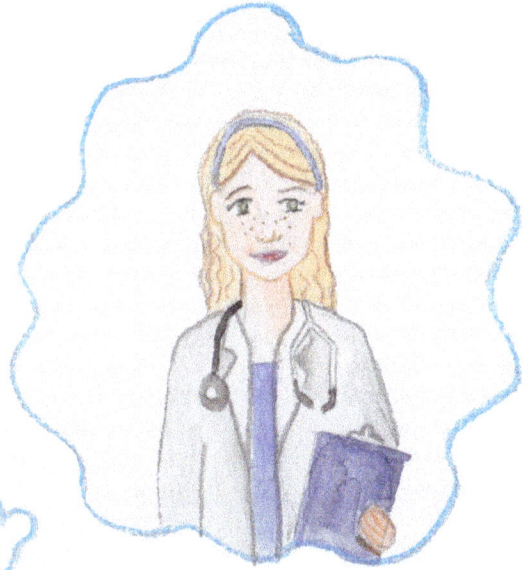

The Pencil & The Paintbrush

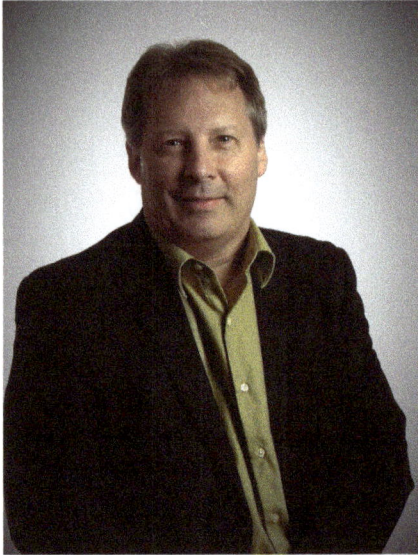

The Pencil

Joseph J. Swope has had an award-winning career in public relations spanning more than 30 years, including managing a statewide childhood literacy initiative between UGI Utilities, Inc. and Reading Is Fundamental. He has also published Pleasant Valley Lost.

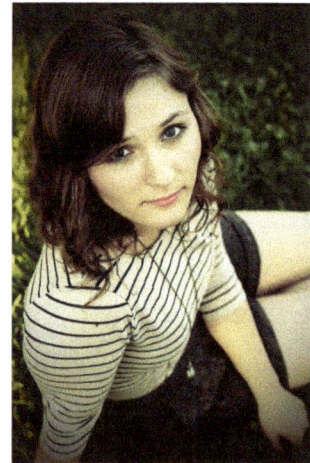

The Paintbrush

Chandra Swope, Joe's oldest daughter, received her Bachelor of Architecture degree from The Pennsylvania State University and worked as an Architectural Designer in Philadelphia, Pennsylvania before her recent move to London, UK.

BLACK ROSE
writing™

www.ingramcontent.com/pod-product-compliance
Lightning Source LLC
Chambersburg PA
CBHW040926050426
42334CB00061B/3476